Dealing With
BABY ECZEMA
Natural Methods That Work

By
Audrey Lynn

http://EczemaFreeNaturally.com

Dealing With
BABY ECZEMA
Natural Methods That Work
Copyright 2013
Authored by Audrey Lynn
ISBN-13: 978-1484844342
ISBN-10: 1484844343

Table of Contents

Copy Right & Disclaimer

A Word From The Author

What you need to know before you start reading this book

The day my son was finally free of eczema, we celebrated. We danced and sang from one end of the house to the other. It was over. After losing so many battles, we'd finally won the war. The monster under the bed was gone and the Bogey man in the closet was banished to Never Never Land forever.

I remember every battle of that war too, as if it all happened only yesterday. I remember how helpless I felt watching my son scratching and crying himself to sleep every night and then, waking up in the morning to find him tangled in his bloody sheets. So I truly understand how every parent feels watching helplessly while their child suffers with eczema.

At one time, I had a very promising career as a college lecturer. But it soon became clear to me that there was no one in my family or community who could properly care for a baby with eczema, so I gave it up to be able to stay home and care for my child myself.

Over the years, I had spent thousands of dollars looking for remedies for this horrible condition, something that would ease the itching and heal my son's broken skin. I tried creams, medicines, tests, and anything anyone suggested, but nothing seemed to work for more than a day or two. Then the eczema would be back, with a vengeance.

But, I persisted in my search. How could I not? Day after day, I watched my son suffer. There had to be a reason for this and I knew if I found the reason, I might just be able to find a cure, or at the very least, relief from the symptoms.
Now, after taking a step back from all the doctors and the well-

meaning advice of friends and family, and after many long days and nights of research, I finally understand what it takes to cure eczema, and as I said, my son and I have celebrated our victory over this terrible skin disorder.

I'm sure you have heard from everyone you have turned to for help, that there is no known cure for eczema. Well, I beg to differ. That is only partially true. And understanding this disorder is the first step toward healing it. That's what this book is about, helping you to understand eczema and helping you to find ways to help your child.

Taking care of a child with eczema is stressful, to say the least. I felt isolated and lonely because no one else around me could understand what I was going through trying to help my child cope with this disorder.

As you're reading this book, I want you to understand, and to know, you are not alone. I know what you're going through. But most importantly, I want you to know that you are not to blame for your child's eczema. Have faith that you are doing the best for your child and you will be able to conquer this condition, too.

This book does not offer any instant miracle cures for eczema, but instead, it will help you to understand why eczema happens and how you can help your child overcome this condition using his or her own body's immune system to eliminate the allergen.

One dilemma many parents face is deciding whether to seek medical treatment or take the natural route to treat their child's eczema. This book will discuss the natural remedies I used to help my son win his battle from eczema. While I am a strong advocate of natural remedies, though, there are a few things you need to keep in mind.
One important thing to remember is that, while the remedies I

mention in this book worked for my son, they may not work for your child. Once you have read this book and you understand the basic reasons for eczema, you will understand that each child's immune system reacts differently to different potential allergens.

It is important to know the basics, such as **nutrition and proper skin cleansing**, and start from there to determine what works for your child. Understanding the basics is critical, as this is when healing can begin. No matter what remedies or treatments you give your child, without knowledge and understanding of the basic causes of eczema, your attempts at healing will be futile.

Taking the natural route toward healing takes time, and many parents give up and turn back to using antihistamines and steroids because they can't bear to see their child suffer. Steroids seem to be the miracle cure, giving their child the relief they so desperately need. However, bear in mind, **THIS IS NOT A LONG TERM SOLUTION**. Steroids simply treat the symptoms; they will not cure the condition. Even though the natural route takes a longer time to see effect, the result is PERMANANT. And your child will not be dependent on steroids for the rest of his life. Isn't that worth some sacrifice on your part?

Be persistent and use the suggestions in this book as a guideline to help you in your quest to find remedies for your child.
And last, but not least, have faith in yourself.

I hope you will enjoy reading this book as much as I enjoyed writing it.

Audrey Lynn

Special Thanks To...

Lucie Nunez, a qualified naturopathic practitioner with a Diploma in Holistic Nutritional Practice, for sharing her experience and story with me. Lucie's baby girl had severe eczema since birth and she has successfully cured her baby from eczema without using harmful steroids and antihistamines.
I also would like to thank the mothers who would like to remain anonymous for sharing their experience and resources with me.

Chapter 1

Baby Eczema

An Introduction

When we become parents, we assume the responsibility of raising another human being. We not only assume that responsibility, we welcome it. And we don't just raise that child like it is a vegetable or a puppy. We care for that child, we shelter it, provide food, and warmth, and more love than we ever dreamed possible. We share our hopes and our dreams with that tiny baby each night when we are rocking them to sleep. And we do everything within our power to keep that child safe, warm and happy.

We can check under the bed for the Bogey man and leave the closet light on to scare away the monsters. We can put kisses on scraped knees and pinched fingers and grab tiny hands before they dart out into traffic. The inequities and wrongs that they suffer on the playground, we can usually erase from their memories with a hug, or if that doesn't work, a lollipop from the special jar in the cupboard.

But some of the "bad things" that creep into our children' lives are beyond our power to control. Some "owies" can't be healed with a kiss. And some monsters won't go away, no matter how many lights you turn on or how many lollipops you throw at them.

When our children are sick with the flu or the sniffles, it is one thing. Yes, we have a sleepless night, or two, or maybe even three. We even spend time wondering what we did wrong. Maybe we should have put a hat on them, or maybe we shouldn't have let them stay up so late. We worry and fret until the fever breaks and the tears stop. But we know, in a day or two, the worst will have passed, and life will go on. And it does. And everything is rainbows and lollipops again.

But for the parent of a child who has eczema, there is no end in sight. Their child is in agony almost every single minute of the day. And they don't miss just one night of sleep, or two, or even three. It is every single night. Every single night they have to worry that their child is scratching himself raw while he sleeps.

The Eczema Monster

That "Monster" is Eczema. 1 in 10 children in America is diagnosed with this disease, and only 4 out of every 10 children who have it will grow out of it. Doctors estimate that 65 percent of eczema patients are diagnosed in the first year of life and 90 percent of patients are diagnosed before the age of five.

Eczema is a skin disorder which causes the skin to become itchy, red, painful, and swollen. Scratching can make the skin bleed. It can also make the eczema worse. Sometimes, the skin becomes thick and scaly. It generally begins in childhood and some children are even born with it, or it appears shortly after birth. Often, the symptoms fade as the child grows but some will have it for life. In fact, it is estimated that 30 million Americans have eczema: 1-3% of adults, and 10-20% of children. Of the total number of children with eczema, 70% of them started when they are younger than 5 years. 60% of these children with eczema continue to have one or more symptoms in their adulthood.

Eczema typically affects the insides of the elbows, the backs of the knees, and the face. But, it can cover most of the body. Now imagine, your 6 month old infant has this horrible disease and their poor little body is burning and itching. And if they do have the motor skills to scratch, all they are going to do is make it worse. They tear up their skin and actually leave open wounds. But scratching doesn't do anything except make it itch and burn even more.

The most common type of baby eczema is atopic dermatitis. The common symptoms include itchiness, dryness, redness, and inflammation of the skin.

The other common type of baby eczema is infantile seborrhoeic eczema, also known as cradle cap. This condition commonly affects babies below one year. The exact cause of cradle cap is not known. The good news is this type of eczema is not itchy and does not cause discomfort or pain to the baby. This will clear up in a few months.

Basically, there are 2 causes for eczema in babies and toddlers.

Firstly, their skin barrier, which is supposed to keep the skin moist does not function well. Thus, their skin gets dry easily and allows irritants to get in easily. Besides the skin, the immune system for babies with eczema tends to react strongly to irritants that gets into their skin, resulting in red and itchy skin. The following chapter will take a closer look at these two causes and how to deal with them.

But before that, we look at the effects of conventional medication to cure eczema in babies.

Chapter 2

Conventional Medical Treatments and Potential Side Effects

If you are reading this book, it probably means you have already sought medical treatment and advice from at least one doctor, and you are not satisfied with the results. This is generally because all your doctor is doing is treating the Eczema symptoms, and not treating the root cause of the problem, which is your child's weakened immune system. Let's take a look at some of the current treatment options prescribed by physicians.

Topical Steroids – *Despite their potential side effects, steroids remain the number one method for controlling eczema safely and effectively.* The type of steroids normally prescribed for treating eczema is cortisone creams or corticosteroids. For children, the commonly prescribed steroids are Hydrocortisone, which contains 1% of steroids. Doctors will usually comfort parents that the mild steroids content will not do any harm to children.

However, that could be deceiving as we look at the possible side effects on using steroids on children.

Growth retardation
Infections
Skin Rashes

Skin Irritation
Thinning of the skin
And this is just a partial list!

You might be wondering how an ointment or cream, which is applied to a rash on your child's arms or legs can cause growth retardation or skin thinning.

Our skin is the largest organ of our body and one of the side effects of using topical steroids to treat childhood eczema is that it causes your child's skin to become thin. This allows the steroids to be absorbed through the skin and into the bloodstream, where they then affect your child's normal growth. These topical steroids can also cause skin discoloration, and with some children, the skin develops marks similar to stretch marks.

This list of possible side effects is not limited to children, and adults may have even worse problems. It is important to note, too, that these side effects can begin appearing in as little as 4 months from the start of steroid use, especially in children whose skin is much thinner than an adult's to begin with.

As I stated above, because our skin is porous, when we apply ointments and creams, especially to dry skin, our skin absorbs then and they are passed through to the bloodstream.

Now, can someone please explain to me why we are risking our children's health, and perhaps their very life, by exposing them to the harmful side effects of steroids? And why we are doing it if all we're going to accomplish in the end is ...***controlling the eczema safely and effectively, and effectively manage the condition?***

If we're not going to CURE the disease, but only try to MANAGE it, why are we taking such HUGE risks?

That is exactly what you should be asking your doctor. Of course, he won't be truthful with you. He won't tell you he is pushing that cortisone so he can afford the boat he just bought or that he's putting his kids through Harvard on your buck. He won't tell you that if he does take care of whatever it is that's causing your child all of this pain and agony, and then he wouldn't be able to send you a big, huge bill every month!

Here's another "treatment" that may be prescribed by your doctor:

Elidel - *The following information is from* Elidel.com *– their own website!*
"Elidel is a prescription cream for people ages 2 and older who have mild to moderate eczema. Learn how Elidel can *control the itching and redness of eczema.*"
And this....
The safety of using Elidel cream for a long period of time is not known. A very small number of people who have used Elidel cream have had skin cancer or lymphoma.
And THIS!
The most common side effects are a feeling of warmth or burning where applied, headache, cold-like symptoms such as sore throat and cough, and rarely, *viral skin infections*. Limit sun exposure during treatment, *and even when Elidel is NOT on your skin.*

Now, just to really drive my point home, the point being that your doctor doesn't care if he ever finds a cure for your child because then he'd have to actually work like the rest of us to earn a living. Pardon the strong language here, but this is true in the medical industry. Here's another one, which is frequently prescribed to manage Eczema:

Protopic – The following information is from Protopic.com – their own website!

   "WARNING: The safety of using Protopic, and drugs like it, for a long period of time is not known. *A very small number of people who have used Protopic have had cancer (for* _**example, skin or lymphoma).**_ However, a link with Protopic has not been shown. Patients should avoid using Protopic continuously for a long time and _**apply Protopic only to areas with eczema**_. If the eczema does not improve within 6 weeks, patients should talk to their doctor.

Protopic should not be used by patients who are allergic to any of its ingredients. The most common side effects with the use of Protopic are stinging, burning, or itching.

And This!

Patients should avoid natural or artificial sunlight (sun lamps or tanning beds). Patients should not use Protopic if they have a skin infection on the area of skin to be treated. The skin being treated should not be covered with bandages, dressings, or wraps.

And THIS!

Only your doctor can weigh the risks and benefits and decide if Protopic is right for you. Please see the Medication Guide and talk to your doctor if you have any questions."

My son started using topical steroids at birth. Because of my ignorance, I continually used that for 2 years. Only when I noticed my son was slower in terms of physical and mental development, did I know I had made the biggest mistake in my life in giving him alien drugs for 2 years, just because his doctors said so. The longer your child is given steroids, the longer it takes to heal eczema. These drugs are toxins, and the body needs to get rid of the toxins before healing can begin. So, do not repeat the same mistake I made.

Listen To Your Child's Body ...

When there is something wrong with our bodies, we show symptoms of illness. When we have the flu, the symptoms are fever, headache and nausea. The symptoms are our body's way of telling us something is wrong and our immune system is working overtime to cure it. We can take medicines to relieve the symptoms – aspirin for the fever and headache and Pepto for the nausea, but we still have to wait for the virus to run its course through our body. By taking over the counter medications, we haven't gotten rid of the virus (root of the problem), we only suppress the symptoms. To be totally healed, your immune system has to work hard to fight the virus. If you have a strong immune system, you will win the battle.

The above can be applicable to eczema.

The manifestations of eczema, the red, inflamed skin, the itchy rash, the swelling and pain, are all signs that something is wrong with our body and that our immune system is unable to handle it. We can suppress the symptoms, or even temporarily eradicate them, by applying these steroid creams and ointments. But, it still doesn't do anything to address the fact that there is something wrong inside our body and our immune system can't handle it. And once we stop using these creams and ointments, the symptoms will reappear because we haven't addressed the real underlying problem.

That is why steroids can suppress the eczema symptoms, but once we stop applying it, the eczema comes back. Then, we apply bigger doses of the cream to suppress the symptoms. Then, they reappear with a vengeance after we stop using the medication and now you need to use even more steroids to suppress it. This is a never ending cycle, isn't it?

Instead, what we should do is help our child's body to fight eczema. And the first step is to listen to your child's body, and how you can work with your child to fight eczema.

But before you go into that, if you ever need to take your child to see a doctor, please read below.

Pediatric Dermatologists

Trust me, I know there will be times when you feel it is necessary to take your child to see a doctor. Don't beat yourself up about this. Even your most diligent efforts may not be enough to keep a serious infection at bay. The fact that you're trying natural methods to treat your child's eczema doesn't mean you can't seek medical attention whenever you feel it is necessary.

But, if you do choose to consult a physician, it is best to see a qualified Pediatric Dermatologist. A Pediatric Dermatologist is better educated in treating childhood skin disorders and will be more qualified to properly diagnose and prescribe treatments. If your child's skin has become infected, a pediatric dermatologist will be better equipped to assess the situation and prescribe the necessary mild antibiotics.

Do not bother to waste your time going to a general practitioner or even a pediatrician. I have seen many of them and if I had listened to them, my son will be still using steroids till this day.

For more information, and to find a Pediatric Dermatologist in your area, you can visit The Society For Pediatric Dermatology website.

If you really need to use steroids...

If your child is having very bad flare up, and you feel you need to use topical steroids to control the condition, do not feel bad about it. Natural remedies take time and in time, when your child is under tremendous suffering, use topical steroids if you feel you need to but with caution.

Please follow the instructions carefully. Steroids, no matter how mild they are, cannot be used for a long period of time. Depending of the type of steroids you are prescribed, the maximum duration you can use is 2 weeks on average. Another thing is do not apply steroids on large area. You should always apply on small area of the skin only.

Remember, too, that these topical steroids are not a long term solution. You should only use them as a temporary solution while you continue to work on helping your child fight eczema naturally.

So what actually causes eczema in babies? Depending on how you feed your baby, the causes of baby eczema may vary.

Chapter 3

Eczema in Formula Fed Babies

When it comes to what triggers eczema, no one, not even the medical doctor has the definite answer. I have spent a good amount of time consulting with various doctors. I also went straight to the horse's mouth for my information – mothers of children with eczema.

In my book, **Cure Child Eczema**, the main cause of child eczema (2 years and above) is his weakened immune system, which makes him more susceptible to allergens and accumulate toxins in the body. However, for babies, as their immune system is still developing, the cause of eczema is somewhat difficult to ascertain.

For formula fed babies, the main cause is most probably the formula as that is the only source of food for the baby. It is worth investigating what formula suits your baby best. If he has milk allergies, switching to soy based formula may be the answer. Check with your baby's doctor for any recommendations of soy formula. Enfamil soy formula is commonly recommended. If your baby has both milk and soy allergies, then the next best alternative is Nutramigen, which contains highly hydrolyzed protein that reduces the chances of a reaction.

Make sure the formula you choose does not cause constipation. If the formula is not promoting regular bowel flow, you may want to consider changing it. When the daily toxins are not released through the bowel track, toxic releases through the pores of the skin will result an eczema flare up.

Probiotics play an important role in healing eczema in older children and adults. However, recent studies have shown that babies with eczema can indeed benefit from formula supplemented with prebiotics.   (http://www.webmd.boots.com/children/news/20130328/prebiotics-in-baby-milk-may-protect-against-eczema)
Alternatively, look for probiotics for infants. You can then add it into the formula. Take note of the correct amount to be added.

Finding the right formula is unique to each baby, so you need to be patient and find the right one for your baby. Besides formula, your baby may be allergic to his surroundings. Please refer to Chapter 6 for a list of non food allergens.

The next step is to establish a skin care routine (Chapter 7). Once your baby is ready to start solids, read Chapter 5.

Chapter 4

Eczema in Breast Fed Babies

If you are breastfeeding your baby, congratulations on your decision to give your baby the best food in the world. Breastfeeding is best for babies with eczema. It is recommended to breastfeed your baby for as long as possible. DO NOT LET ANYONE TELL YOU OTHERWISE, including your baby's doctor. I am sure you have heard stories of mothers who are forced to stop breastfeeding after being told her baby is allergic to her breast milk!!! There is nothing worse than depriving your baby of the best food in this world! In fact, you can actually help heal your baby from eczema by giving him the essential nutrients that can help his body fight eczema via your breast milk.

Is Your Baby Allergic To Your Breast Milk?

As the baby's digestive and immune systems are still immature, the eczema is a sign of food allergies or intolerance. Therefore, it is important for mothers who are breastfeeding to avoid any foods that might cause the allergies. Yes, the allergen can be transferred via breast milk and cause a reaction in your baby. Keep a food diary; start with one group of food at a time. Watch for your baby's reaction. Bear in mind that reaction may not happen immediately. In some cases, reaction will only show up in 4 to 7 days later. A diary is very useful as you can track back to what you have eaten few days ago after the reaction happens.

To identify the food allergen, you can start with this 6 types of common foods that make up nearly 90% of the foods that people are typically allergic to.

Milk, Eggs, Soy, Peanuts, Fish, and Wheat.

The best way to narrow it down and determine which is the problem food for your baby is to completely eliminate all 6 items from your diet for 3 weeks. Then, reintroduce each food one at a time, back into their diet to see which one is causing the allergic reaction. To make things easier, keep a food diary and note down the date and food eaten as well as your baby's reaction.

If none of the 6 types of food above is responsible for your baby's eczema, then consider eliminating these foods listed below. You should eliminate them one by one and note down the reactions. You need to eliminate a type of food for at least 1 to 2 weeks to more accurately determine the allergen.

The following list of foods should be used as a guideline:

Strong acid producing foods

Remove strong acid producing foods like beef, chicken, and pork from your child's diet for at least 90 days. There are two types of foods, acid and alkaline and an ideal diet should be 75% alkalizing foods and 25% acidifying foods. Our bodies work best when the internal environment is at 7.00 pH, which is just to the alkaline side of neutral. If we consume too much acidic food, the body must neutralize this acid in prevent the blood from becoming too acidic.

The body neutralizes this acid with the alkaline foods we eat. But if the balance is off to begin with, then it has to extract that alkaline from surrounding cells, which causes them to become diseased.
Animal flesh has a high concentration of uric acid, which closely resembles caffeine. Initially, we feel pretty good after we eat a high protein diet. But over time, this excess acid builds up in our bodies and the toxins then begin to affect the cells. The immune system then has to work overtime to rid the body of these damaged cells and eventually, it becomes overworked. One exception is fish. Although fish is also an acid producing food, it also provides some valuable nutrients if it's eaten just every once in a while, especially oily fish. Fish is a good source for strengthening bones with its high content of essential fatty acids, calcium, and vitamin D. **Essential fatty acids are important nutrients for the health of your skin.**

Grains that are considered high-glycemic foods
These include corn chips, instant processed grain mixes, cakes, pies, pastry, processed breakfast cereals, instant grain cereals, white rice, and white flour pastas.

Vegetables From The Nightshade Family
Nightshades or *'Solanaceae'* refers to a group of vegetables or fruits that are toxic to the human body. *'Solanaceae'* are known to possess alkaloids that are toxic to humans. The toxins in these vegetables are known to attack the nervous system, joints, brains, and even cause cancer. They are also inflammatory, and because eczema is also inflammatory, it makes sense to avoid them in your child's diet unless you are absolutely sure your child is not allergic to them.
The major nightshades include:
potatoes (not sweet potatoes)

tomatoes
capsicum
eggplant
strawberries
sweet and hot peppers (including paprika, cayenne pepper, and Tabasco sauce)
What many people do not realize is that these seemingly harmless foods are causing their illness. The foods are so common and most of us are raised eating them, and will never suspect they are harmful to us.

Yeast bread

Instead of yeast bread, serve whole rye bread leavened with lactobacillus. Also, try unleavened breads that contain no flour, yeast, sugars, or oils and only include the fiber and germ of the whole grain. These usually contain some combination of sprouted spelt, millet, flax, oats, kamut, amaranth, or quinoa.

Hydrogenated oils and margarine

These foods are so altered they are not even considered real foods. Instead, use oils made from flax seed, hemp seed, walnut, safflower, sunflower, pumpkin, sesame, almond, or olive.

Refined sugar

Eczema can be a form of internal yeast infection and sugar aggravates the condition. The symptoms of eczema disappear in some children after refined sugar is removed from their diet. Sugar can be hidden in cereals, fruit juices, prepared foods etc.

Even ready made baby food has too much sugar.

Artificial sweeteners

Artificial sugars are chemical additives and man made substances. **If you must use a sweetener, use organic unprocessed sugar cane.**

Non-food

Such as salt, alcohol, regular and decaf coffee and tea, regular and diet sodas, artificial sweeteners, preservatives, food colorings, additives and man made supplements. Also, remove enriched flours. 'Enriched' means synthetic vitamins and minerals have been added.

Junk Food and Processed Food

If your diet includes instant noodles, canned food, and other junk food, it is time to throw them away. Instant foods like instant noodle soup and microwave pizzas, fast food like fries and greasy burgers, potato chips, candy, sodas...all of these foods contain levels of preservatives and chemicals that are harmful to your baby's immune system.
You will have to get in the habit now of reading ingredient labels before you buy. Many foods that are promoted as organic foods or health foods have hidden ingredients you should avoid. If it turns out that your baby is allergic to eggs, even the smallest trace of egg in a loaf of bread could cause a flare up.

Doing the elimination diet should allow you to identify the allergen. However, if you still unable to do so, you can see a

Pediatric Allergist. Do a test and determine the food your baby is allergic to and eliminate that from your diet.

Boosting Your Baby's Immune System, And Yours...

As food allergies are a major cause of eczema flare ups, many children with eczema are not eating a wholesome diet because they have to stay away from certain food groups. I remember when I used to feed my son only rice and carrot because he seemed to flare up after eating most types of food. However, staying away from all possible allergens also meant my son was not getting the nutrients he needs for his body to be strong. Needless to say, my son's eczema did not get better, even when I eliminated all possible allergens in his diet.

The main key to fighting eczema is a **strong immune system**. Good nutrition is essential to a healthy immune system. As the only food source for your baby, it is essential that you include foods that can help boost the immune system and are beneficial in fighting eczema. Your baby can then receive these much needed nutrients via your breast milk. The following is a list of foods that are known to fight eczema:

Foods That Helps Fight Eczema

Essential Fatty Acids And Vitamins

Essential fatty acids (EFA) and Vitamin E aid in maintaining the moisture in the cells of the skin. This is important because the skin's moisture barrier serves as a protective barrier against free radicals. Omega-3 and Omega-6 fatty acids can be found in fish, flaxseed, soy oil, canola oil, hemp oil, chia seeds, pumpkin seeds, sunflower seeds, leafy vegetables, and walnuts. Another source of Omega-3 fatty acids is found in cold water fish like tuna, salmon, and sardines.

Minerals

Magnesium rich foods are important to those who are prone to allergies. You can include these magnesium rich foods in your diet : spinach, sunflower seeds, pinto beans, tofu, and halibut. Another essential mineral is zinc. Some studies have shown that people with eczema are zinc deficient. Zinc rich foods include tofu, beef, lean ham, chicken, and crab.

Probiotics

Probiotics mean *"for life"*. They are living microorganisms, which provide health benefits far beyond basic nutrition. They can relieve lactose intolerance and prevent allergies and many types of infections. Probiotics are basically the opposite of antibiotics. They contain beneficial bacteria and they support digestion by breaking foods down for absorption by the body. Prebiotics are food that encourages the growth of healthy bacteria. They do not contain live bacteria like probiotics.

Recent studies have shown that probiotics and prebiotics can help relieve skin disorders like eczema and psoriasis. Probiotics should be taken with food or shortly after eating. Studies also show that giving probiotics and prebiotics to babies in their first year in life strengthens their immune system and thus, helps to reduce chances of allergies.
The best way to give probiotics to very young babies is via your breast milk.

Alternatively, look for probiotics for infants and put some on your nipple during breastfeeding.　If you are expressing your milk, you can easily add it into the bottle.

Grape Seed Extract

Grape seed extract is an industrial derivative of whole grape seeds.
I started to notice the benefits of **grape seed extract** after reading a book called, <u>What Your Doctor Doesn't Know About Nutritional Medicine May Be Killing You.</u> This is a great book.　I am always of the opinion that you shouldn't believe 100% of everything your doctor tells you.

As a result of its high concentration of antioxidant and flavanoids, grape seed extract is helpful in fighting skin disorders such as psoriasis and eczema.　As a natural antihistamine, grape seed extract may help control the sneezing, congestion, and other symptoms of allergies.　Working together, the antihistamine and anti-inflammatory properties can keep allergic reactions like hives, hay fever, and eczema at bay.

Chapter 5

Starting Solids For Babies With Eczema

It is recommended that you only start introducing solids after 6 months of age. You can start with introducing low allergenic fruits and vegetables as first foods.
Low allergenic first foods include:
Apple
Pear
Sweet Potato
Parsnip
Carrots
Courgette
Cauliflower
Grains such as rice and quinoa

Fruits and vegetables should be steamed and pureed. Choose only organic fruits and vegetables. To prepare rice or quinoa, you can simply simmer in water till tender and soft.

As for those high allergenic foods such as eggs, gluten, fish, dairy, soy, celery, nuts, tomato, berries, and citrus, it is recommended that you introduce them after baby is one year old.

When Introducing A New Food

When trying a type of new food, you should start by giving a tiny bit (a teaspoon). Note down the type of food and the date you introduce the
food to your baby. Then, wait 4 days. If there is no reaction, then you can give that food regularly (once or twice a week).

Only introduce one food at a time, so when your baby has a reaction, you know which food cause it. However, do bear in mind that reactions can occur days AFTER the food is eaten. In my son's case, his eczema flared up 4 days after taking the trigger food - cocoa. It took me a long time to identify the culprit. What helped me was the food diary I kept. Therefore, it is very important that you note down what you have given your child. And make a list of the foods he is allergic too.

You have to also bear in mind that, the reaction might be caused by other factors. If your baby seems to react after taking a certain food, take that food off his diet for a few weeks. Then reintroduce the food and see if it is really the trigger. If your baby's condition does not show any difference after the food is taken off for a few weeks, then check the non food trigger. For a list of non food triggers, please refer to chapter 6.

What About Supplements?

For babies, strengthening their immune system will take time. Introducing vitamins, green vegetables and water as they grow will gradually boost their immune system. Keep your baby's diet simple and natural. Avoid any processed food. A strong immune system will help your baby to fight eczema as he grows.

If you think your baby needs a boost in his immune system, then you can introduce infant multivitamin in liquid form to supplement vitamin deficiency. Also, supplement your baby diet with ¼ teaspoon of organic spirulina (mixed with water) every morning and evening.

Chapter 6

Common Non Food Allergens

The following is a list of the many allergens that are known to produce eczema flare ups. Although it is by no means a list of everything you need to watch out for, it is a very good place to start. The best way to help your child is to try to eliminate anything that will cause an allergic reaction.

Dust Mites

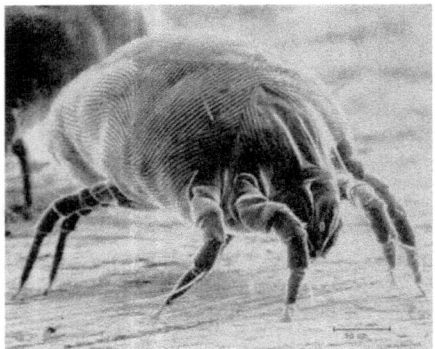

House dust mites live in moist, damp environments and feed on flakes of shed human skin. They are so small you can't even see them and they love to hang out in places like your bed and pillows, your furniture, soft toys, and carpets. Many people are extremely allergic to dust mites, whether they suffer from eczema or not.

Steps to take:

- [ ] **Use a dust mite cover for your mattress**
- [ ] **By a latex mattress that is mold and dust mite resistant**
- [ ] **Use a non-toxic, hypo-allergenic pillow**
- [ ] **Get rid of carpets and have wood floors**
- [ ] **Vacuum regularly with an allergen filter attached**
- [ ] **Use a damp cloth when cleaning surfaces**
- [ ] **Wash bedding regularly in hot water**
- [ ] **Avoid furry toys and soft furnishings**
- [ ] **Keep your house well ventilated**

Pets

Many people have an allergy to animals and it has been found that contact with furry animals can increase the risk of developing eczema.

Avoid having contact with animals, especially the furry kind

If you have a dog, shampoo him regularly

Try removing your pet to another home for a while to see if the symptoms improve

Keep your house free from fur and dust

Chlorine Water

If your baby feels itchy or his skin feels extra dry after a bath or shower, it could be the result of chlorine or other toxins in your tap water. You probably need to install a good water filtration system in your entire home. I have readers who wrote to me that installing a good water filtration system is all they needed to heal their child's eczema. If it is not possible to install a water filtration system in your home, boiling baby's bath water is a good way to get rid of chlorine.

Household Cleaning Agents

For babies', chemical household cleaning agents can be toxic to their delicate skin. Do not use chemicals in and outside the house if possible. Avoid using strong bacterial sprays to keep the house free of bacteria. Find natural ways to clean your house. There are a lot of information on this on the internet. Just do a search on Google. You will be surprised to learn that ordinary kitchen ingredients such as baking soda, lemon juice, ketchup, rice, coffee and vinegar are great cleaning agents.

Teething

Eczema may flare up when the baby is teething. Teething is stressful for babies and the excessive drooling will cause eczema flareups. During teething period, use a clean cool damp cloth to clean the salivated area around the mouth. Moisturizing that area frequently should be able to control the flareup.

Clothing

Make sure your baby wears only pure cotton as any other type of material will aggravate the eczema. Some babies are allergic to polyester which is common material in babies clothes. Wool is another common allergen. If your baby is allergic to detergent, then use only mild soap to wash her clothes. Make sure your baby does not get overheated to minimize itching.

If you are having a hard time (who doesn't?) stopping your baby from scratching, you may want to check out Scratch Sleeves at http://www.scratchsleeves.co.uk. The creators of Scratch Sleeves originally made for this for their 4 month old son with infantile eczema and it worked amazingly well. So they have decided to share their creation with other parents.

The other website you need to check out is a store specialized in Eczema Clothing for children and adults http://www.eczemaclothing.com/.

Laundry Detergents

Laundry detergent plays another big role in eczema flare ups in more ways than you think. For one thing, allergic reactions can often bring on a flare up. The overwhelming scent of some laundry detergents is often all it takes to produce an allergic reaction. Think about it the next time you walk down the detergent aisle at the grocery store and you get a headache from the smell before you even get to the end of the aisle.

Laundry detergents can also cause flare ups because they leave a residue in your clothes each time you wash. Residue comes from anything in the detergent that will not rinse out of your clothes after they are washed. And after just 8 washings, it has been found that these residues will account for up to 2% of the garments weight. These residues left on the clothes are potential skin irritants, which can cause flare ups and are found in detergents that include fragrances and brighteners.

This residue does not only irritate the skin, but they also make your fabrics stiff. You can take care of this problem by using a fabric softener, but then you have another residue being left in the fabric which might cause an allergic reaction or be an irritant to the skin. Chlorine bleach is another potential irritant that should be avoided.

Side Note:

it is important to include some more in-depth information here about the difference between soaps and detergents.

People have been making soap for thousands of years by combining fats or oils with alkaline substances, such as ashes or soda ash.

Detergents, on the other hand, have only been in existence since about 1930. They really came to the forefront after World War II, when the war-time interruption of fat and oil supplies, as well as the military need for a cleaning agent that would work in mineral-rich sea water and in cold water, had further stimulated research on detergents.

Detergents are non-soap washing and cleaning products that are created from a variety of chemicals, synthetic products, and petroleum. There is nothing natural at all about detergents and your child could be allergic to any one of the myriad of chemicals used in their production.

You should also be aware that not only do detergents leave residue on your clothes if you use a laundry detergent, as opposed to a laundry soap, but there are detergents in shampoo, toothpaste, dish detergents, dish washer detergents, all of your household cleaning products. There are detergents in places you never even dreamed of. And detergent residue is present on nearly every surface of your home.

Check the ingredients on the liquid hand soap you use. Chances are; it contains detergent. You now have detergent residue on your hands. The same can be said for your dish soap. Even your toothpaste.

For an amazing account of how one family was finally able to eliminate all traces of detergents from their home and almost completely cure their son of eczema, visit SolveEczema.org. If you, like this family, have tried everything you can possibly try, to eliminate allergens from your child's environment, yet he is still suffering from horrendous flare ups, it is quite possible detergents are your culprits. It won't be an easy task to completely eliminate them from your home, but it is well worth the effort if it heals your child.

Please note, too, a flare up after coming into contact with an allergen may not always be immediate. It can sometimes take up to 2 weeks for your body to react to an allergen you have been exposed to. That's why it is so important for you to keep a diary of everything your child eats or comes into contact with.

Metal Poisoning

If you've addressed all the possibilities of food allergens and environmental and external allergens, you may want to consider the possibility of a metal allergy. Metals such as nickel, mercury, lead, etc., can get into the body and promote toxic poisoning. Children can be exposed to these metals through inoculations and immunizations or even from breast milk from the mother. If you suspect your or your child might have metal poisoning, consult with your physician for testing.

Vaccination

This is probably a controversial topic. There are increasing numbers of babies reported to have chronic eczema after their routine vaccination. There are some cases where the parents reported that their baby's skin were normal prior to taking the vaccination.

By taking a vaccine shot, your child's immune system is seriously compromised. Once the immune system is weakened, your child's body becomes vulnerable to various allergens and thus, triggers an eczema reaction. Besides the weakened virus, a vaccination shot contains other dangerous substances such as mercury. If your child has allergies and skin problem, vaccination can worsen the condition.

Moreover, vaccinated children are more prone to various allergies compared to those who are not vaccinated.

However, to vaccinate or not, this is a decision parents have to make. I am not qualified to give any advice on vaccination. I have no way to tell that vaccination caused my son's eczema. But if I knew at that time the potential dangers of vaccinations, I would have thought twice before giving my son the shots. Or, I would have delayed the vaccination schedule until my son is much older. Anyway, for me, it is too late now. But for you, vaccination is one topic you need to look into before making the right decision for your child.

Chapter 7

Establishing A Good Skin Care Routine That Keeps Eczema Away

It is especially critical to establish a good skin care routine for babies with eczema. It is very important to keep the skin clean, and equally important to moisturize to keep the skin as supple as possible to prevent breaks and tears. Natural, organic skin care products that work with the skin to promote healing are the best choice. Synthetic products, like the ointments and steroid creams prescribed by your doctor, are seen as foreign allergens by the body and will cause more harm than good.

You may have heard that baths should be reduced as not to dry out the skin. I have tried giving my son a bath once in two days. His eczema did not get any better. Instead, the itch got a lot worse. Imagine not washing your hair for a few days... It is the same scenario. Therefore, I do believe baths is necessary to keep the skin clean as the skin releases harmful toxins via the skin. If the skin is not clean, this will build up and encourage bacteria growth. So, go ahead and bathe your baby everyday!

Is The Water In Your House Laced With Chemicals?
You need to check the water in your home. Depending on where you stay, the tap water in your home may be heavily chlorinated. Chlorine may be one of the reasons for eczema flare ups if your child is allergic to it. One mother wrote to me that her son's eczema is completely gone after she installed shower filters in her home. And that is the only thing she did. So, I do recommend installing a water filtration system in your home

for chlorine free water for drinking and showering. However, if installing a filter is not possible, you can boil the baby bath water first to let chlorine evaporate.

A Proper Skin Care Routine

One of the biggest reasons people fail to get their eczema under control is because they fail to establish a skin care routine. You can't take care of your baby's skin whenever you have time, or whenever you remember to do it. It has to become a part of your and your baby's day to day life and it's much easier for both of you if you establish a routine.

You are going to have to spend a lot more time on skin care than the average parent. So if you get a routine set, it will just become part of your day and you will be more apt to stick to it. And if your baby knows that bath time comes at the same time every night, followed by moisturizing, eventually it will become part of his daily routine too, and he will even start to look forward to it.

When choosing skin care products for your baby, it is important to make sure the product is not adding to the damage of their sensitive skin. Always start with ONE type of skin care product and note if there is a reaction. If so, then switch to another product. If you try a few products at a time, you would not be able to identify the culprit. It is important to eliminate possible allergens in your baby's skin care routine. Avoid using shampoos, soaps with chemicals, bubble bath etc. Look for natural and organic skin care products without harsh chemicals. You will be surprise what alien chemicals are commonly added in children's skin care products.

Here is a list of harmful chemicals to look out for:

Triclosan (similar to Agent Orange, a pesticide)
Sodium Lauryl Sulfate, Sodium Laureth Sulfate (SLS) (used in garage floor cleaners and engine degreasers)
Parabens
Ureas (release formaldehyde, weakened immune system)
Synthetic Colors (usually labelled as FD&C or D&C, followed by a color and a number)
Diethanolamine (DEA) (linked to cancer)
Propylene Glycol, Propylene Oxide, Polyethylene Glycol (weakened skin cells and linked to cancer)
Synthetic Fragrance (avoid any product with fragrance as an ingredient unless derived from essential oils or other natural sources)
1,4-Dioxane (Avoid synthetic ethoxylated ingredients, including those with myreth, oleth, laureth, ceteareth, any other "eth," PEG,
Polyethylene, polyethylene glycol, polyoxyethylene, or oxynol, in their names)
Ethyl Alcohol (Ethanol)
Benzalkonium Chloride (BAC) (linked to cancer and known to cause allergies)

Do take note that some "natural" commercial soap or shampoo may not be as pure as many such products still contain SLS. I buy my son's skin care products from a local organic store, where they make their own organic soap using coconut and palm oil. You may want to check out your local health food store in your area. Many of these stores may make their own soaps and shampoos and sell at a much lower price.

Moisturizing After Bath
Immediately after the bath, follow up with a good, natural moisturizer. By doing this immediately following the bath, the skin is still moist and the moisturizer seals that moisture in.

As soon as your baby is out from the tub, blot off – DO NOT WIPE – excess water with a clean, dry towel and liberally apply moisturizer while the skin is still damp (within 3 minutes). This helps seal that additional moisture into the skin and traps the moisture absorbed in the bath.

There are many natural moisturizers. It is very important to remember, when choosing skin cleaners and moisturizer, choose products that are fragrance free. Products that have fragrance also contain alcohol to carry the fragrance and the alcohol also has a drying effect on the skin. I use virgin coconut oil for my son with great results. However, coconut oil may not be right for your baby. So here are some alternatives, which I have received great feedback from parents who have used the following products. Remember to try a small amount to ensure your child is not allergic to the oil. If you see a reaction in your child, do not continue. Try another alternative.

The following natural ingredients promotes natural healing process of the skin. Look for product with these ingredients.

Vitamin E oil
Aloe Vera
Ginseng
Oatmeal
green tea
champhor
echinacea
calendula
Almond oil
Borage oil

The following skin care products have received positive feedback from parents:

Arbonne Baby Products have received great feedback from

parents. This product has no phthalates, no mineral oil, and no animal products. Arbonne Baby Oil is great to use for cradle cap.
California Baby Calendula Cream
Aveeno Oatmeal Bath
Un-petroleum Jelly

Remember, what works for other babies, may not work for your baby as each baby is unique.

Chapter 8

Conclusion

It is really challenging for mothers to cope with infant eczema especially when they have not had eczema before. I remember being blamed by my mother-in-law for eating all the wrong type of food during my pregnancy, which caused the eczema in my son. Of course, that made me feel very bad and helpless. The last thing you should do is feeling guilty. Think positive. You have a healthy and beautiful baby. That is the most important. Eczema is not some kind of fatal disease or a handicap. Being positive makes a whole lot of difference.

The most important thing to remember is that eczema is not an incurable disease. You may have to try different dietary combinations and different skin care combinations until you get just the right mix. But when you do, flare ups will be completely eliminated, naturally, and your child will have the quality of life every little one deserves. Remember this; your baby's eczema may get worse before getting better. This is because of toxins in your baby's body being released through his skin. So this is something to keep in mind before you give up on natural healing and call it a bunch of crap.

Last, but not least, the journey in healing eczema can be long and difficult with a lot of tears. I have been on that road and saw light at the end of the tunnel. So, never give up helping your child heal eczema. Have faith in yourself. Many parents have successfully healed their baby without using drugs, so can you.   You just need to be persistent. Keep trying until your baby is free of eczema. Your child deserves an eczema free life, and your owe your child that.

Bonus

Please visit this link to download your bonus reports :

http://www.curechildeczema.com/getbonus.html